Introduction to the Methods of Grigori Grabovoi

"General Deliverance and Harmonious Development"

Svetlana Smirnova
and
Sergey Jelezky

Jelezky Publishing
www.jelezky-publishing.com

First English Edition, January 2012

© 2012 English Language Edition
SVET Center, Hamburg
Svetlana Smirnova
www.svet-centre.eu

First English Edition, January 2012
© 2012 English Language Edition

Sergey Eletskiy, Hamburg (editor)

English Translation: Margarete and William Mieger

Cover Design: Sergey Jelezky
www.jelezky.com

ISBN: 978-3-943110-35-7

For further information contact:
SVET Center, Hamburg
www.svet-centre.eu

According to the responses we have received, the contents of this book have helped many people. We are confident that this will continue to be the case.

Nonetheless, we would like to point out that the techniques of Grigori Grabovoi are mental methods for the guidance of events in one's life. These methods are dependent upon one's personal spiritual development. Because we are dealing with topics relating to one's health, we give this express notice that such influence is not a "therapy" in the conventional sense of the word and is therefore not intended to limit or replace professional medical care.

When in doubt, follow the directions of your doctor or a therapist or pharmacist whom you trust! (When following conventional methods, you must expect to geconventional results.)

Jelelezky Publishing/SVET center, Hamburg

Disclaimer:

The information within this book is intended as reference material only, and not as medical or professional advice.

Information contained herein is intended to give you the tools to make informed decisions about your lifestyle. It should not be used as a substitute for any treatment that has been prescribed or recommended by your qualified doctor. Do not stop taking any medication unless advised by your qualified doctor to do otherwise. The author and publisher are not healthcare professionals, and expressly disclaim any responsibility for any adverse effects occurring as a result of the use of suggestions or information in this book. This book is offered for your own education and enjoyment only. As always, never begin a health program without first consulting a **qualified healthcare professional.** Your use of this book indicates your agreement to these terms.

Table of Contents

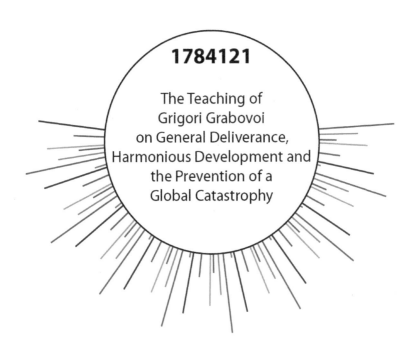

1784121

The Teaching of
Grigori Grabovoi
on General Deliverance,
Harmonious Development and
the Prevention of a
Global Catastrophy

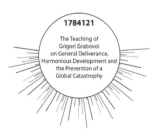

1784121

The Teaching of
Grigori Grabovoi
on General Deliverance,
Harmonious Development and
the Prevention of a
Global Catastrophy

Human!

You are the world, you are eternity.

You possess immeasurable powers.

Your possibilities are limitless.

You are the embodiment of the creator.

In you, his will resides,

through his destiny you change the world.

In you, his love resides.

Love all life as he does, he who has created you.

Do not embitter your heart. Think good, do good.

Good will return to you with longevity.

Love will give immortality,

faith and hope, prudence.

With faith and love

your invisible powers will come alive.

And you will achieve all that you dream of.

Immortality, it is the face of life.

Just as life is the trace of eternity.

Create to live in eternity.

Live to create eternity.

Grigori Grabovoi

Preface

Dear Reader,

For already more than 11 years and with much success, we have concerned ourselves with the teachings and the corresponding methods and technologies of Grigori Grabovoi. In 2010 (English Language Edition – 2012) we published our first booklet, "Methods of Healing Through the Application of Consciousness," (ISBN:978-3-943110-34-0) which has given many people a first impression of these teachings.

We bring the current work, "Introduction to the Teaching of Grigori Grabovoi," as a continuation of this work with the goal of furthering your knowledge of these valuable teachings. As before, we are concerned here with the basic humanistic view of "the deliverance and harmonious development of the inner and outer worlds." With these words Grabovoi challenges us to rethink our positions in order that we become the driving force on Earth, the protector of the Biosphere and the conditions needed for life for all living beings – for the sake of the prevention of catastrophes.

The teaching of Grigori Grabovoi tells us that every person can become the captain of his fate by actively guiding the events in his life – including individual and collective health – by means of his soul, spirit and consciousness. Teaching how to do this is the purpose of our seminars and literature. In the practical aspects of this work we are not so much concerned with meditation as with the development of a conscious focus, the ability to actively give our attention a specific direction in order to master a task we have set ourselves, or that motivates us, or that has been given us from a higher source. One aspect of every task is always the general well being of all elements of the universe, for the quality of our thoughts when working with the "Norm of Creation" will accelerate – or retard – the attainment of personal results.

On a universal scale there is only one goal: eternal and infinite development of our consciousness of the boundless love of God, whose creation we are and whose qualities we also can and should develop in thought and deed. When we understand this, then we will also understand that everything always happens for us in the best possible way. Grigori P. Grabovoi writes: "Our life task consists of translating the knowledge of the soul into a meaningful form of expression and applying this consciously."

Knowledge, which comes from the Creator, is needed to accomplish this! All of the methods of deliverance, of self-restoration and of the guidance of events in one's life that Grigori Grabovoi offers mankind are founded upon the unique understanding that he has received from the Creator. This he has phrased in the terminology and concepts of modern science. "But Grabovoi has not only developed methods for the deliverance of mankind. His greatest accomplishment is, through a researching of the subtle realms, the establishment of a new definition of the laws of these realms. The subtle or ethereal world is unknown to many scientists, but one can work with this world when you have knowledge of its laws." (See also: W. J. and T. S. Tichoplaw, "The Teachings of Grabovoi, Theory and Practice, Part 2.") In his book "Applied Structures of the Creative Field of Information," Grabovoi describes how man is organized (created). Here he also describes how man through his spiritual nature stands in direct relationship and interconnection with the entire universe (external reality).

Through an understanding of this spiritual interrelatedness, one comes to see that every person is directly and inseparably connected with the entire world and brings forth an effect (a change) in it through his thinking, feeling and actions. In like manner an effect (a change) in the external world also leads to a change in the inner reality of man. If we now take our consciousness into account, all unpleasant events – including diseases – are "lessons" that we must learn in order to structure our consciousness for the successful realization of the task of God: the eternal, harmonious unfolding of reality.

For a better understanding of the not always simple methods of Grabovoi, we have published this second booklet to support you in the successful realization of your personal tasks. It should help you to better learn the methods and techniques and to be able to successfully apply them for yourself or others. Ideally, one can also employ these methods in a preventative manner or in the sense of a positive goal orientation for one's personal health of body, soul and spirit, thereby actively supporting in an individual and general sense the deliverance and harmonious development of the whole. We are pleased to accompany you along this path!

With heartfelt regards,
Svetlana Smirnova and Sergey Jelezky

SVET- Center, Hamburg
Private Academy for the Human Being

The Teaching of Grigori Grabovoi on Deliverance and Harmonious Development

The teaching of Grigori Grabovoi, "General Deliverance and Harmonious Development," encompasses general deliverance as well as the deliverance of each person individually. It is concerned with securing eternal, creative and harmonious development. A focal point of this teaching is the actual prevention of a possible global catastrophe.

"The practical realization of my teaching is based upon the student directing his actions by means of conscious decision to the deliverance of all beings and to the prevention of a global catastrophe and through this also resolving his personal issues." In this process the consciousness encompasses any chosen event and its creative guidance. This means: the more you use the methods and technologies of the teaching of Grigori Grabovoi for the deliverance of everyone, the better the resolution of your own issues. This is why, when you make use of and spread the teaching of Grigori Grabovoi, your desired result manifests in the fastest possible manner due to the law: "Anyone who acts on behalf of everyone receives from the Creator his due." (Grigori Grabovoi, "Foundation Course for the Structuring of Consciousness")

The entire universe consists of objects of information. It is a very complex information system. Information plays a basic role in the life of every person. Every living being on Earth exists from the moment of their birth until the end of their life as objects of information in an informational field. Life on Earth would be impossible if the life forms on it were not able to receive information from their external environment, if they did not understand how to process it and use it and pass it on to other objects of information.

Everything in the world is interconnected through informational ties. For this reason if you change something on this essential level, the whole system can be changed. Grigori Grabovoi developed a method for the conscious control of informational systems. The core concept of this method concerns the influencing of the informational system of a person through consciousness and perception. Grabovoi says that the total volume of information consists of the information of matter, of consciousness and of the external environment. And according to the law of conservation of information, a change in the magnitude of information of a particular form creates a corresponding change in the magnitude of information in the rest of the forms.

Man is an informational object and thus a disease is also an informational object. Any particular situation represents a set of informational objects and their interrelationships. A person with his mental capacity, which is capable of creating any and everything, can create any specific informational object, imbue it with the needed qualities and characteristics and, through it, operate upon and with the external informational field. In short, man has in general the capacity to direct and guide the course of events. In this regard it is important to mention that we continuously exercise a certain – subconscious – control over information. It is precisely this guiding activity that delivers us from catastrophes and cataclysms (very large, devastating destruction). When a person combines his personal tasks with the global task of the deliverance of all, then a transition occurs from controlling action on the physical plane to exerting an effect upon the system of thought. As in the technology described here, thought itself becomes the agent of control.

– Question to Grigori Grabovoi: What is a disease?

A disease is the lack of correspondence between one's desires and needs with one's existing tasks in the world. Disease must be considered under the aspect of harmonious relationships in the world. When somewhere and somehow harmony is disrupted, discomfort ensues.

– Grigori Grabovoi, what is your understanding of health?

Health is a condition of reality in which the relationship between man and the external world is in the greatest possible harmony. But health is not only a physical condition. It is also a moral as well as a social and even political phenomenon. Health is a system of relationships in which the healthy body exists. (G.P. Grabovoi, "The Technologies of Deliverance," Interview with Grigori Grabovoi.)

In the course of our seminars we are compiling a reference list of the terms used in Grigori Grabovoi's books and seminars and also in works about him. This terminology list helps one to correctly understand the information presented. The meaning of such key concepts as "soul," "spirit," "consciousness," "perception" and "physical body" have been taken from the books and lectures of Grigori Grabovoi. These entries are concerned with core concepts, whose true meanings are hardly to be found in the dictionaries of this and the last century.

Soul – The soul is that "substance" made by the Creator for eternity. It is an eternal element of the world. The soul is steadfast and unshakeable. It exists as a part of the innate structure of the world and is therefore the foundation of such further concepts as "spirit." And so it is possible from a certain perspective to say – the activity of the soul is spirit. And so you can say that when you perfect yourself spiritually in the sense of a creative development in the world, you can change the soul. One principle of revivification is that eternal life has the necessity of soul development as a prerequisite. And in fact, in the life eternal – according to the development of a person and the society – all tasks are created anew and new tasks are created. The development of the soul is absolutely necessary if a person is to adequately master these new challenges. The soul is a personal accomplishment of the Creator – it is the light of the Creator (of Creation). The soul exists in that certain "absolute" space, in which God, the Creator, created it.

Consciousness – Consciousness is a structure that allows the soul to direct the body. The soul, whose material component is the body, acts upon outer reality through the structure of consciousness. In the broadest sense consciousness is a structure that unites the spiritual and material worlds. Through a change in consciousness spirit is also transformed and with it our actions, which means: because the soul is a part of the world, it is present in every event that takes place. A change in human consciousness thus creates a change in all other elements of the world. The development of man, his perfection, is connected to the development of his consciousness. Mankind's primary task consists, therefore, in changing his consciousness and in climbing to ever higher states of awareness.

The Kingdom of God – A key term in the New Testament is the "Kingdom of God." The Kingdom of God is first and foremost a higher state of consciousness and the advancing to ever higher states of awareness is the stairway to heaven. Here we find the meaning of

16   ©2011 Copyright Grigori Grabovoi, Svetlana Smirnova, Sergey Eletskiy

the text "The Kingdom of God is within you." For if the "Kingdom of God" is a higher state of awareness, then it is also within us. And when Jesus repeatedly says "awaken," then he means this literally, because our normal waking state is in comparison with this higher consciousness only a deep dream state, comparable with daydreaming and with dreaming while asleep.

True consciousness – True, higher consciousness is a state of awareness, which reflects the reality of the world in an infinite time/space continuum. This form of consciousness makes it possible for us to live forever in a process of eternal development. True consciousness is a true and precise reflection of the system of the development of the world, as it exists within infinite time and space. It includes the holographic principle of the reflection of the whole in every part. True consciousness develops along with the development of the spirit. It is important not to forget that even the tiniest cell is connected with the entire macrocosm. And changes on the micro level can, according to the law of general relationships, transfer over to the macro level.

Expanded consciousness – Expanded consciousness is a state in which perception is expanded and begins to encompass the entire domain of consciousness.

Perception – Perception is that portion of consciousness, an instrument of control, through which subjective reality is projected into individual consciousness.

Matter – Matter is past consciousness.

Concentration Exercises
and the Guidance of Events through Information
for the Restoration of the Norm

The concentration of one's consciousness can lead to radical change in the structure of the entire world. With the help of focusing one's consciousness, for example, on some organ of the body, it is possible to change the condition of this organ, to restore its health.

The ability to concentrate one's consciousness grows greater and greater according to the spiritual stature of a person, according to the degree of his development and self-improvement. In this context the concentration of consciousness refers to an increase in the information density, i.e. more information within the same unit of space.

When in the course of development a person's concentration of consciousness reaches a certain level in a particular space, then this space begins to subjugate itself to this person. This results in a change in the structure of the world: the world no longer determines the structure of man, but now man sets the tone.

When the concentration of consciousness becomes greater than the concentration of matter, for example an automobile, then a person becomes invulnerable. He becomes indestructible. The thoughts, words and deeds of a person become the primary element; cars, buildings, planets and other material objects become in contrast secondary elements. This is the next level of existence.

This is precisely the reason why I am passing on this knowledge, so that after adopting this new system, people can progress to the guidance of worlds. This will be a completely different level of existence. Here there will no longer be any decay, here completely different processes will take place. They will be processes of the renewal of worlds, that is processes by which the eternal gives birth to more eternity, by which the state of one eternity passes into the state of the next eternity.

This results in an enormous compression of consciousness, through which the speed of information exchange is greatly increased leading to completely different structures in the end result: structures of the highest state of consciousness, structures of the highest form of life. On this level thought and deed are synonymous.

Grigori Grabovoi

- Our consciousness possesses immense creative powers; creative activity and control of the physical body happen by means of consciousness, and our soul is hereby the structure that directs everything.

- When one begins to work with the techniques for the guidance of events, you need to activate all inner resources to the maximum.

- During a period of concentration, you must continuously hold the goal that you want to accomplish in mind. This goal could be the manifestation of a desired event, including the removal of a disease.

- Prepare yourself mentally to create the events that you need in the same manner as the Creator does.

- While focusing, attempt to feel how the light of your soul, streaming in a bright ray from your third eye, illuminates the object of your concentration; this increases the effectiveness of your guidance of events.

Concentration on Numbers, Working with "Restoration of the Human Organism through Concentration on Numbers"

Numbers are not only mathematical symbols, but also energies of the Creator. Working with a single number or a sequence of numbers can bring about a healing. You can, for example, select a number sequence from the book by Grigori Grabovoi, "Restoration of the Human Organism through Concentration on Numbers" (ISBN: 978-3-943110-14-2) for its corresponding disease. Put the number sequence into a sphere and then mentally reduce the sphere to the size of a match head. Now take the healing vibrations into your body and hold them there for a while.

It is also possible to picture the numbers and number sequences in various qualities of light and various colors. All concentration exercises are to be carried out in a state of inspiration, which means that you must enter into the state of the spirit.

Normalizing Body Weight

1. Mentally place the number sequence **4812412** (obesity) into a small sphere.
2. Compress the sphere into a point and mentally place it into your abdomen.
3. Now place the number sequence **1823451** (endocrine and metabolic disorders) into another small sphere and mentally place it into your hypophysis.

Restoration of Vision

First Variation:

1. Mentally place the number sequence that regulates vision **1891014** (eye diseases) into a small sphere.

2. Compress the sphere down to the size of a tennis ball and mentally place it in your head.

3. Take off your glasses and picture the sphere emitting beams of silvery-white light like a floodlight shining out of each eye.

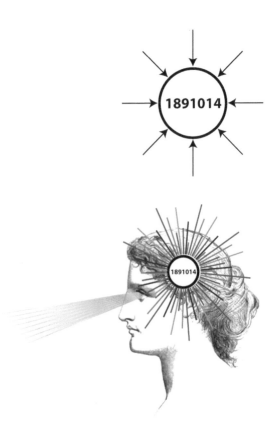

Second Variation:

Mentally place a deliverance cell (see "Creation of a Deliverance Cell") – regardless of the nature of your eye problem – into your eyeball and let the deliverance cell multiply in a clockwise direction.

The deliverance cells provide the diseased cells with information as to the Norm, which then contributes to the restoration of normal vision.

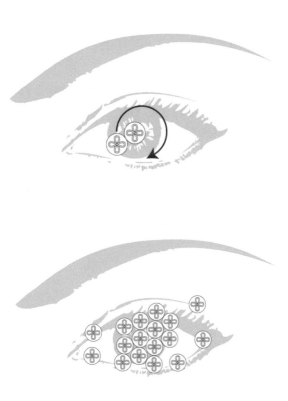

Technologies for Rejuvenation

Focusing on a Photo:

Take a photo of yourself in which you are young and happy. Hold it in front of yourself at eye level. In the space between your face and the photo, on the level of your forehead, picture the following number sequences, and focus on them:

2145432 and **2213445**

You can also illuminate the number sequences with a silvery-white light. If it is easier for you, you can write the two number sequences on the photo – above your head. While concentrating upon the photo, remember the happiest moments of your youth and your present time and imagine happy moments for your future. You can repeat this exercise several times a day until it has become anchored in your consciousness.

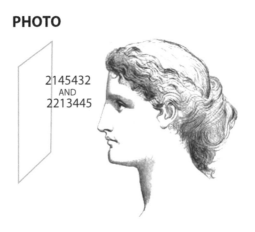

PHOTO

2145432
AND
2213445

Focusing on Plants:

1234814   and   1421384

Mentally place each number sequence on the leaf of a tree or a plant or on the branch of a tree. Mentally place yourself to the right of the plant in the physical form in which you like yourself the most.

This concentration exercise uses the method of reflection. The purpose is the following: You start by concentrating upon a plant. The plant can exist physically as it appears in external reality. In this case during your focus, you can simply look at the plant. Or you can visualize the plant. Here, focus on the shape of the plant. While you are concentrating on the selected plant, picture how the light that is reflected from the plant begins to form your desired result. Even better, do not just imagine this event, but rather see it in front of you as a "real" event. You construct the actual event in front of yourself. One advantage of this exercise is that the constructed event becomes harmonious for in our world the plant already lives in harmony.

Focusing on Stones:

8275432   and   8223745

Mentally project these number sequences onto stones and picture an image of yourself in which you are healthy, young and happy.

Concentrate on crystals or stones. You can even take just a grain of sand for this focus. Let's say you have selected a particular stone.

Now imagine a sphere around it as you are focusing on it. This is the information sphere. Mentally see how all of the events that you need appear within this sphere. You simply place the events you need into this sphere.

(from Grigori Grabovoi, "Concentration Exercises," ISBN: 978-3-943110-31-9)

Methods for Working with Numbers

Regardless of the situation we are dealing with, we speak of the "Norm." But what is this Norm? It is important to always recall: the Norm is a harmonious development, the general deliverance, a state of eternity and a state of love according to the Norm of Creation (the Creator).

Technology 1:
Concentration on the Number 1, Squeezing a Result Out of a Number

1. Picture a number of your choice as a spatial form (for example the number 1).

Now mentally write into this number the information about an event, a result or a goal that you wish to achieve.

Next press this structure from all sides into a point. This compression process squeezes out the desired result and it appears in your reality.

2. If visualizing is difficult for you, you can use the following method:

Take a piece of paper, draw a graphic representation of the number and write your desired result inside of the number (see illustration below).

Next squeeze the paper into a ball. The effect is the same: the result is pressed out and manifests itself.

Once the process of "normalization" has been started, the normalizing continues automatically on its own. This is the key!

Ideally, you will do this as the Creator does – once for all time (this is how He made the world). So be aware that you are doing this once and for all!

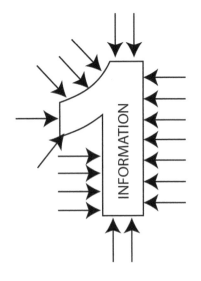

Question: *When we use the number sequences from Grabovoi for various diseases, upon what do we need to focus?*

Answer: *You do not focus on the disease, but on the Norm, that is, that information, which leads to the condition of the Norm (Creation). This already exists inherently in the number sequences, because numbers are themselves eternity and Norm, in other words: eternal life, harmonious development and general deliverance.*

Grabovoi created his teaching on deliverance and harmonious development according to the Norm of Creation and therefore every number sequence carries the information of the Norm within itself. A focus on the sequence is a focus on the Norm!

Technology 2:
The Guidance of Events Using the Number Eight (8)

Divide the number eight into two parts, an upper and a lower (you can do this with any number, but the number eight is optimal), and then place the condition of the Norm of the Creator into the upper portion – and in the lower portion put the accomplishment of a task or goal, your desired result.

To initiate the manifestation of the event, put the following into the lower portion:

- The number **one** (1) stands for **the beginning of the action** (our decision to undertake it) and imbues the event with the power of a positive result.

- The number **two** (2) stands for **the action itself** (our activity in relation to the goal).

- The number **three** (3) stands for **the result of our action** (for the desired result), for an outcome in the sense of the Norm of Creation.

- The numbers **four** (4) to **nine** (9) stand for **the unfolding of events** (obscure processes or imponderables) in relation to our activity. It is possible that in the course of our actions various or numerous steps must be taken in order to reach the desired goal. This is dependent upon the interaction of a person with the process, on inner and outer aspects, on the specific structure of the person and on his life circumstances.

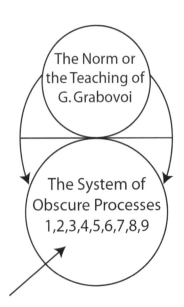

Example: You want to get your driver's license.

In the upper portion of the 8, enter "NORM" (according to the Creation) – without precisely knowing what this normed condition is.

In the lower portion put, according to your desire: (1) want to get my driver's license, (2) for this I must "learn to drive" and "take a driving test" and (3) "I have my license." In addition add the numbers (4) to (9) for further steps that could possibly be connected with your goal. In this way the undefined variables are "discharged" and you go about your task in a relaxed manner.

Technology 3:

Concentration on the Number Three (3)

This technology is based upon the powers of our logical reasoning and a clear perception of reality.

Consciously prepare yourself for the result of an action. You know exactly what result you will get without knowing in detail the steps that lie in between. Know that the number three contains the logical basis of any previously taken action. This puts you in a position to bring any situation to the Norm. The result will at least be one that brings you specific information relating to the desired goal.

Concentrating on the number three creates variations of logical developments. The logic of the Creator intersects with the logic of man in the number three.

Example: You are planning a vacation trip.

Plan your trip to the moment where you have returned healthy and happy back home again – after having had a wonderful vacation – and your life is going on in a positive direction. In other words, focus on a consequential result of your vacation: on the relaxation and a joyful life with new goals.

Methods for the Guidance of Events
Using Colors of the Visible Spectrum

Color is that characteristic, which most closely corresponds to the spiritual aspect of man. This is related to the fact that a color can be perceived as infinitely large. When a person works with colors, he is actually influencing the infinite system of interconnections on the informational level. For man, the "language" of color is a trustworthy instrument of self-knowledge. Our behavior, our condition, our health and our mood are all dependent upon the color spectrum of our environment.

Through the effect of a color upon our organism, that is, through the corresponding frequency, a diseased organ that finds itself in disharmony can be restored to the condition of the Norm.

The core of this method consists of the fact that the color, which speaks to you the most, delivers information. According to the "Teaching of Deliverance and Harmonious Development" by Grigori Grabovoi: Through the selection of further colors in addition to the one first selected, the goal of giving a guidance to reality is realized. It is as if the colors bend harmoniously together. In just this moment the Norm of the event is set.

The Technologies:

Concentration on a Selected Color

Enter a state of concentration and picture a silvery-white column of light to your left side that extends upwards (Fig. 1 below). Mentally connect the light column with the "Teaching of Deliverance and Harmonious Development" by Grigori Grabovoi.

To your right side picture a light column in any other light shade of color of your choice (e.g. gold, lilac, rose). Now mentally place a precisely formulated task or problem (for example, changing a situation) into this column. Name the deadlines and possible variations for the resolution of this problem. Concentrate yourself and visualize both light columns, which extend upwards into infinity where they join together. They become a single beam of light that contains both colors and shines down upon you from above (Fig. 2 below).

"Look upwards and try to see even further to the place where the colors unite in the beam of light that is shining down from above. This means that it has a structure that contains the color of the teaching as well as your own color. And try to fill the space around you with this color (Fig. 3 below), which is as much as saying: after solving your own problem, try also to resolve other people's issues. As soon as you have visualized this color "raining down" from above, you will notice that your personal goal in the guiding of events has been manifested through the macro deliverance, that is, the deliverance of all.

As soon as the light above begins to stream down faster, think immediately of how this knowledge can be passed on. You think concretely of how to pass on the knowledge. This action should be firm and persistent. You should be certain that you have done everything correctly for the solving of your problem. Position the problem to your right side and you will notice that you no longer are perceiving the space around you because you are primarily working within a system of thought."

Grigori Grabovoi

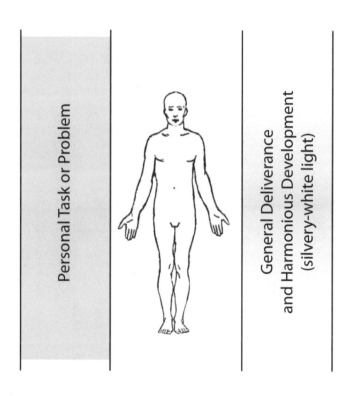

Fig. 1

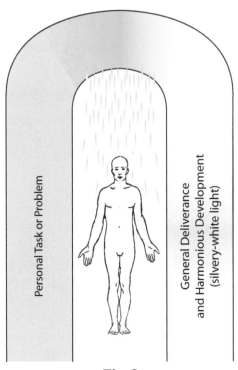

Personal Task or Problem

General Deliverance
and Harmonious Development
(silvery-white light)

Fig. 2

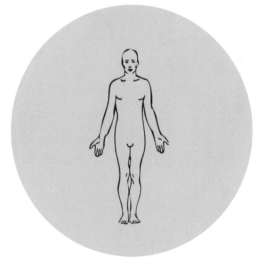

Fig. 3

Concentration on the Colors of the Rainbow

One way to get rid of a disease is by concentrating on the colors of the rainbow. You must work your way through the colors, one by one. Select the color that most catches your attention and focus upon it for 3 to 5 minutes. This color that most attracted your attention will influence its corresponding organ causing it to change the frequency of its vibrations. The color will put the organ into a condition of the Norm. When you focus on a specific color, which you have created with the help of your inner vision, the information of this color is transferred to the diseased organ and this is how it is healed.

"You need to concentrate several times within one hour after 10.00 p.m."

Grigori Grabovoi

Diagnosis with the Help of the Color White

There is an information center within man in which information from the micro and macro levels stands in interrelationship with the cellular level of our body. In every cell certain micro-processes take place that are determined by the functional structure of the cell. The cell and its various parts interact with the entire surroundings.

If the basic cell is divided into a million parts, each part works together with the entire universe and with each part of the organism. Each part of the cell can be divided again into another million parts. As you do this, the impression of a light vacuum arises. It appears as the color white, which corresponds to the original Norm.

The source of every disease, for example tumor formations, is also determined by the light spectrum. When you look at the organism by placing your perception of it in front of the backdrop of the color white, the appearance of every other color is representative of a change in information in the organism. And this change tells us something about the presence and nature of a specific disease. In his original, pristine condition, man has no infirmities. His organism is intact and undefiled. The entire body, all organs, all of the cells of a person are also located in the sphere of information. Disease is a piece of information that comes from without. Somewhere on the outer surface of the information sphere there is an "entry point," where the information of the disease has penetrated the sphere.

The following method is recommended for making a diagnosis:

"Before you lie down to sleep, focus upon your right earlobe and direct your attention to the perception of the color white. Any differentiation from the color white, also in your dreams, which comes without any additional mental effort, can lead to a correction of the disease condition."

Grigori Grabovoi

Through spiritual development, inner disturbances will be reduced.

By selecting specific colors, it is possible to heal oneself, to renew one's strength or to help other people. You will notice how you change or the person you are helping changes. Go to the emotional level and feel how every situation has its own taste, its own smell and its own color. Work with a positive attitude – and your positive vibrations will grow stronger.

Picture one by one the colors of the rainbow. When your gaze is caught by any particular color, then it could be that you need this color right at this moment. Focus on this color for five minutes, let this color pass through you and notice how you feel.

Use this color in your choice of clothing.

This method is very effective. You will notice how its power unfolds if you stay at it long enough.

Guidance of Events Using Sound Waves

Focus upon an individual goal and a collective goal – in accordance with the Norm or the "general deliverance and harmonious development" – and send the information of these goals together with a tone signal of your choice into the universe to be manifested. Tones have electromagnetic characteristics and the sound spreads out in waves into infinity.

Example:
Stand out in nature and listen to the rustling of the wind in the trees. Focus on the above-mentioned goal and send your thought information along with the sound waves, those from the rustling in the trees, branches and leaves that is made by the wind, into the universe.

The information of our thoughts spreads out and works with "infinite" power in the universe for the restoration of the Norm.

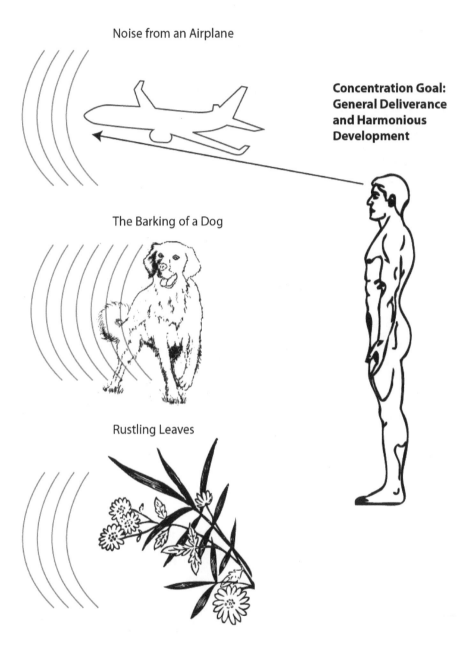

Noise from an Airplane

Concentration Goal:
General Deliverance and Harmonious Development

The Barking of a Dog

Rustling Leaves

Working with Spheres and other Geometric Constructs

The Guidance of Events Using a Double Cone Construct

First mentally construct a double cone (the shape of an hourglass) with a center opening the size of the ring made by putting your thumb and your index finger together. The double cone is positioned horizontally (see illustration below). Now focus on a personal goal and send the information into the right side of the double funnel. At the point where the two cones meet, put the number eight (8) as a symbol of eternity. Intensify the eight by illuminating it with silvery-white light. The information entered reaches the connecting point, is transformed to the Norm and leaves through the left funnel – into reality. The density of the exiting information is the same as the density of the information entered. By means of the eight the transformation becomes lastingly potent. Once the transformation is complete, the construction dissolves automatically.

Right Cone: Entering of events that are to be transformed (disease, pain, unemployment, relationship problems, etc.)

Left Cone: Exit for events that have been transformed to the Norm (health, well-being, satisfying work situation, harmonious relationships, etc.).

Connecting Point: The place of transformation of the information entered to the Norm.

Example: High blood pressure

We see the double cones positioned horizontally in front of us. We place the number eight (8) at the connecting point and illuminate it with a silvery-white light. Next we turn the double cone construct clockwise so that the right funnel is facing our body. We enter the information "high blood pressure" into this funnel ("vacuum principle") and let it move to the connecting point, where it is transformed to the Norm. At the same time we mentally say:

"Restoration of the high blood pressure on a cellular level to the Norm of the Creator."

The information "normal blood pressure" leaves the opposite (back) funnel with the same information density in which it was entered and now it begins to spread throughout the universe.

Double Cone Construct

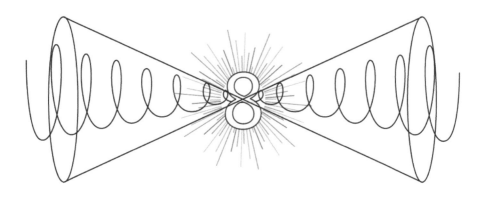

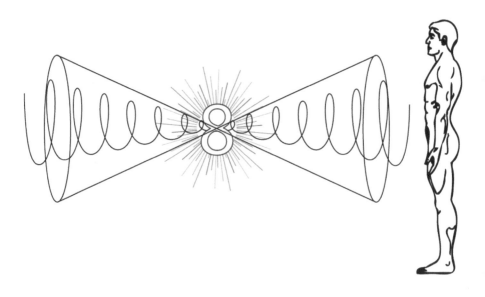

Creation of Deliverance Cells

Picture a number of spheres surrounding your body (see illustration below).
These are defined portions of your mind.

Nearby spheres – **these are the portions of your mind closest to your awareness.**
Spheres further away – **these are the portions of your mind farther from your awareness.**
Spheres still further away – **these are the portions of your mind maximally distant from your awareness** (in the neighborhood of the North Star).

Choose one of these "mind spheres" to be a deliverance cell containing living matter.

Now, one of the mind spheres located farthest (super far) away lights up like a spark. Bring this sphere in closer and start to work with it:
1. Fill the sphere with a silvery-white color.
2. Place the word "deliverance cell" as well as the symbol of eternity (8) and infinity (∞) into the cell.
3. If you have a specific disease, then put the number sequence corresponding to this disease into the deliverance cell. Now let the cell shine with a very bright violet light. The cell is now ready.
4. Mentally put the cell into the diseased organ for the purpose of restoration and move it through the organ in a clockwise direction.

5. Observe how the living deliverance cell begins to multiply and to restore the organ. Picture how the organ begins to emit a violet glow. This is the healthy organ – the NORM. Now see the organ in its natural color (for example, how you would see it in a medical textbook). Anything you do on the informational level – creating something or enlivening something – will then drop to the physical level.

The most effective time for this work is between 10.00 and 11.00 p.m. (Moscow time). In this window of time you participate in the support that Grigori Grabovoi makes available on the informational level.
If you cannot work at this particular time, then move the time window mentally to an earlier point in time. Continue your work until you see that the organ has been restored.

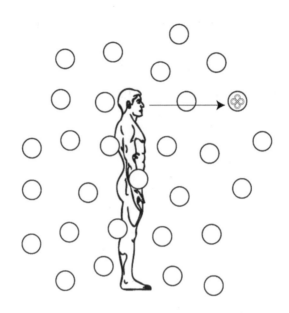

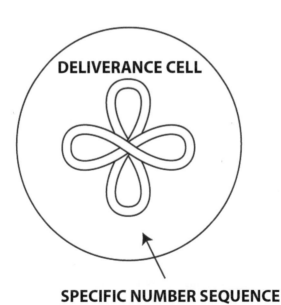

DELIVERANCE CELL

SPECIFIC NUMBER SEQUENCE

Restoration of the Spine

1. Focus on your spine. Along the spine mentally write the word **"NORM"** in letters of light as a support for the healing process in general.

2. Mentally picture a light sphere (Sphere 1 in illustration below) next to your **right hip joint**. Enter the information *"complete restoration of my spine"* into this sphere. Now visualize a brightly shining connection between this sphere and the "Norm" along the spine for the information sends vibrant rays out from the sphere through your body in the direction of the "Norm." (Because problems with the spine are actually always problems of the entire organism, feel how the shining rays fill and thereby restore your entire physical body.)

3. Picture another light sphere (Sphere 2) next to the **right knee joint** and enter in the same information: *"complete restoration of my spine."* There again appears a brightly shining connection between this sphere and the "Norm" along the spine. The bright rays containing the information rise from the knee through the thigh and pass through all body organs on their way to the "Norm" along the spine.

4. Next picture a third light sphere (Sphere 3) next to your right ankle, but this time with the information *"complete restoration of my organism."* This sphere is filled with silvery-white light.

Mentally say:

"Complete restoration of my organism to the Norm of the Creator!"

An intense glow, filled with this information, begins to rise from the ankle, through the calf, through the thigh and up into the body. It takes in the sexual organs, the digestive system, the liver, the spleen, the kidneys and the pancreas. The lungs, too, are completely permeated with this glow. It connects with the "Norm" along the spine and continues to ascend – through the thyroids, through the neck and up into the brain to the **hypophysis**. This organ is so intensively illuminated that a small **silvery-white sphere** appears in the middle of the brain exactly where the skull originally began to form.

5. **A glowing light arch** originating from the right side of your brain passes **into the left hemisphere**. The entire information on what we must do to remain healthy is stored in the right hemisphere.

6. The left hemisphere begins to process the information contained in the light and transfers it to **the entire endocrine system**. This system, which is responsible for the control of our metabolic system, produces the **hormones** needed to completely restore your body and even to rejuvenate it. Your body now functions again according to the **Norm of the Creator**.

7. Enter the actual **time** and **date** and send this information – from this time onwards – into **infinity**.

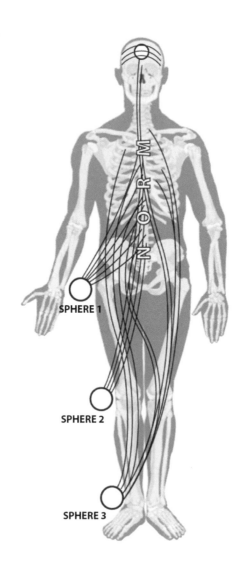

Working with the Spine

Method for Harmonization in Business

The number sequence for the normalization of financial situations is:

71427321893

and the number sequence for the resolution of general situations and problems is:

212309909

To improve your focus, surround yourself with the number sequence: put a copy into your wallet, your passport or some other convenient location. Place the number sequence in your workspace or home.

Method for Resolving Various Situations

- A column of spiritual light exists about 50 cm (20 inches) in front of your body (Fig. 1 below). All of the information about Creation is contained in this column. Say:

"General deliverance and harmonious development!"

- Now make a detailed picture of a situation or a result that you would like to harmonize in your life.

- Place this information in the column, the Light Stream of the Creator, and bend the light stream with the information into a bow, so that the information flows to the midpoint of the bow.

- Now hold the information in your focus for a moment and let it go again by releasing the bow and sending out the information of your desired result like an arrow (Fig. 2 below).

- In this way your information is transported like lightning into reality and transformed into a result.

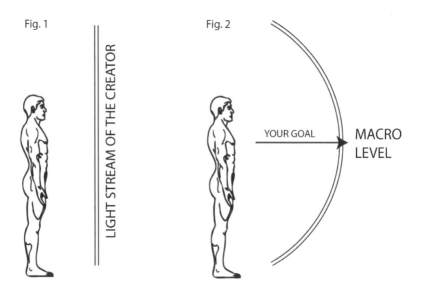

Fig. 1   LIGHT STREAM OF THE CREATOR

Fig. 2   YOUR GOAL   MACRO LEVEL

A Technology for Problem Resolution

All of a person's problems have a point of concentration that is located 2 cm (approx. ¾ inch) in front of the third eye. This is a sphere with a radius of also 2 cm (see illustration below).

In this sphere you find the informational source of the problems. This is the point of contraction for all problems. Some people say that they have a headache because of their problems and rub their forehead at the same time. The process of contraction of a problem does in fact affect the physical structure of a person. But man also has a second sphere, the upper informational center. This sphere, with a radius of 5 cm (approx. 2 inches) and located 2 cm vertically above the head, allows him to have an influence on his problems. It consists of seven segments. The first segment is directed towards the nose. When you connect the information that corresponds to the problem with the information of this segment, the problem resolves itself.

Use this technology when you do not have much time and a quick solution to the problem is important.

This technology not only makes it possible to solve problems, it also helps us to understand their meaning. When you understand why something is happening or has happened, you can reexamine and revalue your actions, thoughts and perspectives.

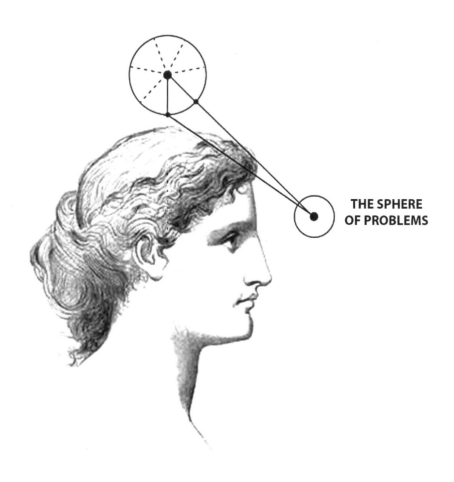

**THE SPHERE
OF PROBLEMS**

Restoration of Paired Organs

1. Stretch your arms out straight in front of you so that the fingers of both hands are pointing to each other and you can see the palms of the hands.

2. Focus first on the index finger of the left hand.

3. Next, with a conscious "impulse" and visual awareness transfer the focus to the index finger of the right hand.

4. Then transfer the impulse further:

> a. From the right index finger to the left little finger
> b. From the left little finger to the right little finger
> c. From the right little finger to the left ring finger.

Try to feel what is happening in your body. You have already achieved a state of spiritual control.

5. Now transfer the impulse to the ring finger of the right hand.

During this exercise new cells are being created, the rejuvenation and/or regeneration of the paired organs has been initiated and the functioning of the brain cells has also been activated and increased.

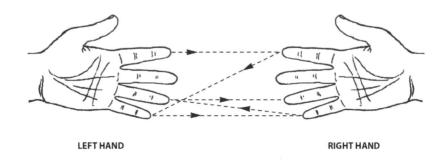

LEFT HAND   RIGHT HAND

LEFT HAND   ## RIGHT HAND

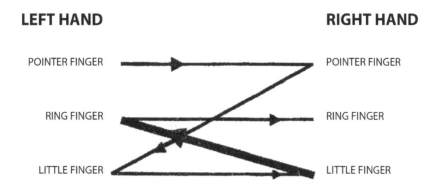

POINTER FINGER ————————▶ POINTER FINGER

RING FINGER ————————▶ RING FINGER

LITTLE FINGER ————————▶ LITTLE FINGER

Diagnosis through Focusing upon
Certain Sections of the Body

The visual "scanning" of the organism is carried out by first mentally dividing the body into 10 separate sections. The sections correspond to the ten fingers of our hands.

Starting with the little finger of the left hand corresponding to the legs and the right little finger corresponding to the head, mentally divide the body into ten sections (see illustrations below).

Next concentrate on the fingers of your hands. Focus upon the finger or thumb in which you first feel a sensation (tingling, heat, vibration, skin reaction, general awareness, etc.). Compare the finger you have located with the illustration and transfer your concentration to the corresponding section of the body.

With further concentration and attention to detail, you can specify a particular organ, a cell or some microelement in this section. The finger that gave you the sensation will also reflect any change in the corresponding body section.

You can use this focus to conduct a diagnosis on the informational level. This concentration exercise can also be done prophylactically once a week.

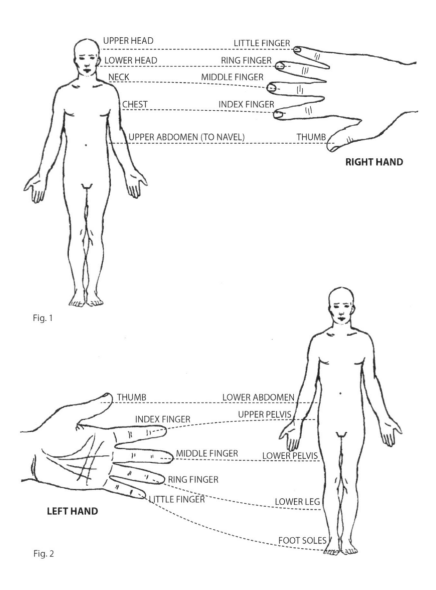

UPPER HEAD — LITTLE FINGER
LOWER HEAD — RING FINGER
NECK — MIDDLE FINGER
CHEST — INDEX FINGER
UPPER ABDOMEN (TO NAVEL) — THUMB

RIGHT HAND

Fig. 1

THUMB — LOWER ABDOMEN
INDEX FINGER — UPPER PELVIS
MIDDLE FINGER — LOWER PELVIS
RING FINGER
LITTLE FINGER — LOWER LEG
FOOT SOLES

LEFT HAND

Fig. 2

58   ©2011 Copyright Grigori Grabovoi, Svetlana Smirnova, Sergey Eletskiy

Method of Protection

The Task of this Method:

The purpose of this method is to transform reality before there is even time for clairvoyance to locate a problem in the future. This means that by working in the system of the "general deliverance…" according to Grabovoi, one should always have the "Norm" or the transformation of information to the "Norm" for every situation that may occur in our life and that we may want to change.

There is a method in working with consciousness that is based upon creating segments of a sphere (1/3 of a sphere), which are able to deflect possible negative information. This means that possible negative information can be "warded off" (deflected) even before its realization.

Description:

- Picture a sphere, for example, in the form of a soccer ball. Mentally divide this soccer ball into three equal parts (see illustration below). The inner surfaces of these segments deflect the negative information.

- Place two of the segments in front of your knees so that the deflecting inside surfaces face outwards.

- An information signal reaches you first at the level of your knees, where you have placed the reflectors. From here you then receive the information, which has been transformed (normed) and sent to the brain.

Explanation:

You reach the future through the movement of your legs and in the motion of the legs, it is the bent knees, which arrive in your future first. This is the reason that information, which always comes from the future, always arrives first at the level of the knees.

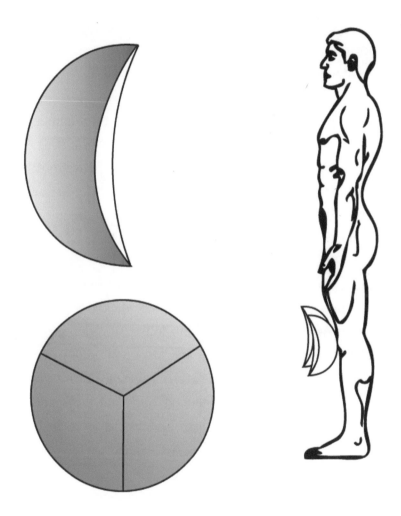

Grigori Grabovoi

Grigori Grabovoi was born on the 14th of November in 1963 in the village of Bogara in the province of Kirov in Kazakhstan. He completed his studies in mechanical engineering at the Tashkent State University (Department for Applied Mathematics and Mechanical Engineering) in 1986.

He is a member of the International Academy for Information as well as the Russian Academy of Sciences. For a time he was a consultant to the Russian Federal Aviation Service and he is the discoverer of and author of a number of works on the Creative Field of Information, which encompasses all informational objects and models in any place on the space-time continuum.

He also discovered methods for the conversion of the information of every action into a familiar geometric form as well as basic principles of remote diagnosis and regeneration. In addition, he possesses a unique form of clairvoyance, of prediction, and has knowledge of numerous methods of therapy. With the help of his clairvoyance, he has "examined" hundreds of airplanes, the space station "Mir" and the space shuttle "Atlantis" for mechanic failure – his observations were in complete agreement with the later findings of the mechanics.

His work is directed toward the prevention of catastrophes through the creation of a non-destructive unfolding of events and he explains how in working for the general deliverance of all, one can come to a guidance of events in the world at large and in one's own personal life.

The SVET-Center
for Spiritual Technologies

Goal and task of the Center: the spreading of the teachings of Grigori Grabovoi on the deliverance and eternal harmonious development of all people.

SVET provides information on the nature of the soul, the spirit and consciousness.

On the basis of the teaching on "general deliverance," technologies are provided for the reuniting of man with the Creator, technologies that lead one beyond all forms of structure.

Spiritual technologies are provided for the understanding of the building of the eternal physical body. Essentially every person can learn these technologies and acquire the ability to pass them on to others.

The Center offers educational courses and health therapy based upon this knowledge.

SVET teaches how to see the divine order underlying the events occurring around us and how to restore your health through your own efforts. For from our point of view, there are no incurable diseases.

Svetlana Smirnova

The neurologist and homeopath Svetlana Smirnova was born in Omsk (Sibiria). She graduated from the state medical college and then worked for ten years as a doctor in the neurological department of the state medical clinic in Omsk. Since 1995, she lives in Hamburg where she founded together with Sergey Jelezky the SVET-Zentrum (Center) for Spiritual Technologies. She teaches seminars and workshops in Hamburg and other places in Europe for interested people from all walks of life.

Sergey Jelezky

After graduating from the College of Technology in Omsk, Sergey Jelezky worked there and later in Hamburg as a professional artist and designer in his own atelier. Together with Svetlana Smirnova, he studied "Geovoyager" (the structuring of consciousness) at "Fond A. N. Petrov," a school for clairvoyance, then at "Hope," the Center for Spiritual Technologies, N.A. Koroleva and W.A. Korolev, and at The Center for Spiritual Technologies "Arigor," I.W. Arepjev (Moscow).

Bibliography

"Concentration Exercises," Grigori Grabovoi
ISBN: 978-3-943110-31-9

Lectures by Grigori Grabovoi

"Restoration of the Human Organism through Concentration on Numbers," Grigori Grabovoi
ISBN: 978-3-943110-14-2

"Unified System of Knowledge," Grigori Grabovoi
ISBN: 978-3-943110-05-0

Notes

Notes

Introduction to the Teaching of Grigori Grabovoi

"General Deliverance and Harmonious Development"

Edition 2012-1,26.01.2012

ISBN: 978-3-943110-35-7

CPSIA information can be obtained
at www.ICGtesting.com
Printed in the USA
LVHW072328140321
681546LV00028B/171